Epsom Salt

The Miraculous Mineral

Holistic Solutions & Proven Healing Recipes for Health, Beauty & Home

Natural Remedies, Holistic Health (Book 1)

by Elena Garcia
Copyright Elena Garcia © 2016

All rights reserved. No part of this publication may be reproduced, stored in a retrieval system, or transmitted, in any form or by any means, electronic, mechanical, photocopying, recording or otherwise, without the prior written permission of the author and the publishers.
The scanning, uploading, and distribution of this book via the Internet or via any other means without the permission of the author is illegal and punishable by law. Please purchase only authorized electronic editions, and do not participate in or encourage electronic piracy of copyrighted materials.

Legal Notice:

This book is copyright protected. It for personal use only. You cannot amend, distribute, sell, use, quote or paraphrase any part or the content within this book without the consent of the author or copyright owner. Legal action will be pursued if this is breached.

Disclaimer Notice:

Please note the information contained within this document is for educational and entertainment purposes only. Every attempt has been made to provide accurate, up to date and completely reliable information. No warranties of any kind are expressed or implied.

Readers acknowledge that the author is not engaging in the rendering of legal, financial, medical or professional advice. By reading this document, the reader agrees that under no circumstances are we responsible for any losses, direct or indirect, which are incurred as a result of the use of information contained within this document, including, but not limited to, errors, omissions, or inaccuracies.

Contents

Introduction-5

Chapter 1 The History of Epsom Salt-10

Chapter 2 Epsom Salt and Your Health-18

Chapter 3: Health Maintaining Tips-25

Chapter 4: First Aid and Epsom Salt-41

Chapter 5: Epsom Salt and Beauty Tips-46

Chapter 6: Epsom Salt in Your Home-60

Chapter 7: Epsom Salt in Your Garden-64

BONUS CHAPTER: Epsom Salt and Essential Oils-70

BONUS CHAPTER: Epsom Salt and Mindfulness-84

Free Complimentary eBook from Elena-95

Introduction

Welcome and thank you for taking an interest in this book. You are about to start a fascinating journey learning about the wonderful world of Epsom Salt. But not only that, you will be learning really easy, practical ways of using them to boost your health and beauty plus some other very unexpected benefits in your garden.

Dig out that packet sitting in the kitchen, or maybe even the garage shelf, that you bought a while ago. It is FULL of the most amazing benefits. If you aren't using Epsom Salt every day, there is something wrong! And the thing that most people tell me when I talk about the benefits of this fascinating power packed powder is 'I never knew you could do THAT with them.'

I shared that lack of knowledge! A while ago I looked at the dusty old packet of Epsom Salt that I'd bought ages ago in a fit of enthusiasm for something I'd read about them on Facebook. I'd apparently used them for a bit and then life took over and I forgot about them. But I must admit, like many people, I was a bit unconvinced that that white powder in the unprepossessing box could actually achieve all the claims that were being made for it. That box had cost just a few bucks and I had the suspicion that something as simple as that and not backed by extensive chemical research by scientists in white coats and coming in at a high price could actually do the job. Boy! Was I wrong!

I should have known better as a lifelong practitioner and user of natural remedies but for some reason I hadn't latched on to this little wonder product. I decided to do something about that and began to do my own 'white coat' research. It didn't take long before I was using them all the time. So in this eBook you will follow in my footsteps for a while before branching off into your own discoveries of this simple homely - but wonderful -product.

I saved money by the bucketload using them as beauty products. I saved time because they worked quickly in starting to support my health

I increased my joy in my garden a hundred-fold because so many plants appreciated the Epsom Salt treatment that they came on in leaps and bounds.

So, anything that's going to save time and money – and works well has got to be worth looking at. Turn to the first Chapter and prepare to be amazed and excited.

The way to use this ebook depends on if you are a big picture person, or whether you like focus and detail. The big picture people should zero in on the first chapter right away. It tells you all about the salts, their history, the various categories of help they can be used for and why they are so beneficial.

After that go to the section you are most interested in and dip in there. Gradually you will read the whole book and have many new ideas about how you can use that dusty old packet in the kitchen cupboard!

The detail people need to zero in on the section that is most relevant to them. Just concentrate on that and start trying out one idea. See if it works for you then move on to the next thing. Once you have been hooked by the Epsom Salt bug you may want to learn some of their history. That can be found in the first chapter. After that you may shift your attention to one of the other uses of Epsom Salt and work your way through that. It always helps to try out the suggestions. Only when you feel the impact in, and on, yourself do you turn into a convert and make sure that Epsom Salt is always in your cupboard and you are using it every day.

Read on and enjoy...

Before we dive into the benefits and uses of epsom salt, I would like to offer you a free gift:

Free Complimentary eBook

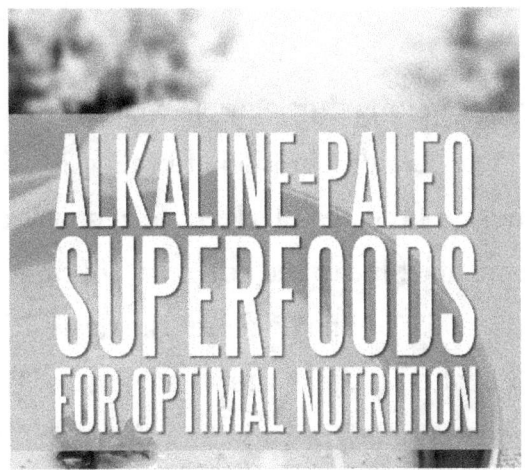

Free Sign Up Link:

www.YourWellnessBooks.com/newsletter

Problems with your download?

Contact us: elenajamesbooks@gmail.com

We're here to help.

Chapter One

The History of Epsom Salt

Once upon a time, a long time ago, there was a little village just to the south of London in England called Epsom. When I say a long time ago I mean a LONG time ago. We are going back in our time machine to the beginning of the 1600's. Four hundred years ago, to a time just after the death of Good Queen Bess (Elizabeth 1), just after the failure of Guy Fawkes in his plan to blow up the Houses of Parliament and about the time when swashbuckling Sir Walter Raleigh, explorer and colonizer of North America, bringer of tobacco to Britain and leader of the expedition to El Dorado in South America was executed. It was a turbulent time in history but through it all the little villages that spread out like plates on a tablecloth all around London went about their business and tried to stay out of the way of politics and war mongering. What they wanted was a quiet prosperous life with their families in the countryside and they went about finding ingenious ways of doing just that.

In pretty little Epsom there was a drought and a local man, Henry Wicker by name, was searching for some water for his cattle. Noticing a small trickle of water filling a hoof print in the meadows around the town he dug down a little hoping to find an underground fresh water spring. On his return after digging he discovered that indeed he had tapped into a small spring that bubbled up from the deep rocky caverns below the earth. Praising the Lord for this gift from Nature he brought his cows to the meadow and stood back to watch them drink. Imagine his surprise when they refused to take a gulp!

Exploring the water a bit more he tasted it for himself and discovered that far from being simple, pure water it was full of minerals dissolved from the rock in the caverns below and then drawn up with the power of the spring. The taste was strong and brackish so it was no wonder the cows had refused it. However Henry had been around a bit and was aware of places like Bath where the Romans had built baths for restoring their health using the hot heavily mineralized spring waters in Somerset. He began to wonder if his little trickle of 'spa' water would have the same properties and help people just as in Roman times.

He tried them out on himself and discovered that he did indeed feel better after a short while. Excitedly he began to bottle the water and sell it to the local people and dreamed of a bustling town rivaling Bath which was being refurbished in an early attempt to bring people in to sip its waters. Later, of course, Bath became very famous in the Georgian 18th Century when the beautiful elegant terraces, crescents, homes and public buildings created by Beau Nash were built to grace the town and turned it into the most desirable resort for the wealthy and high-born society people.

Little Epsom did not have such luck. The spring did not produce enough water for large public consumption although there was a short period where visitors came from as far afield as Cornwall to 'take the waters'. A triumph of good marketing on Epsom's part as the people from Cornwall actually bypassed Bath to travel all the way to the south of London Town!

By the end of the century Epsom was a busy little place with 300 beds for visitors, however the lack of a plentiful supply of the water continued to place a limit on growth. Most visitors stayed for some days, even weeks, and consumed vast quantities of the water in pint mugs. They would drink several pints in the morning then again throughout the day. In the course of a visit they could drink as much as sixteen pints!

Not surprisingly this had a significant impact on their digestion and purging, or detoxing, was the order of the day.

Despite the sinking of a second well on the other side of the town the end of Epsom Spa actually came when the pharmacists in the early 1700's discovered what was in the water that was making it so effective. From the moment that the chemical compound, $Mg_2SO_4.7H_2O$ or hydrated magnesium sulfate, was discovered poor old Epsom was doomed as the salts could now be manufactured and sold very cheaply in powder form. Soon other chemists in other parts of the country were producing the salts too and the chance to make a significant fortune was over.

However, such were Epsom Salt benefits that manufacturing of them has never stopped from that day to this and this is where we in the 21st century come in as we discover what our great, great grandparents knew.

$Mg_2SO_4.7H_2O$ **or Magnesium Sulfate**

What exactly is this?

The formula stands for a combination of hydrated magnesium, sulphur and oxygen which begins to bring us the answer as to why the compound is so effective. Right away we see that Magnesium is a significant mineral within the Salt.

Magnesium

There has been lots of research on magnesium and we know that it is a highly beneficial element in several ways to overall health. In fact it has been called the most important element in nutrition.

Among its many attributes it plays a significant role in heart health. Without it hypertension is likely to get worse and, since heart disease is a silent killer, it makes excellent sense to have your blood pressure taken regularly and if it begins to climb outside your normal range then consider if your diet is deficient in Magnesium. Proper levels of Magnesium also help Coronary Artery Disease and sufficient levels of Magnesium in the body is part of preventing hardening of the arteries and strokes.

Sulfate

The next important element in Epsom Salt formula is Sulfate. Sulfates can only be ingested through certain foods but there are not many foods that give us all the sulphate we need. Fish, organic meat, poultry, free range eggs and grass fed beef are the foods of choice for this purpose. Of course all of these are the most expensive items on a shopping list. It makes sense to have some of these high-quality sulphur carrying proteins weekly. Eating whole grains, pulses and seasonal greens most days of the week with one or two meals of high-quality organic meats will give a good balance.

For vegetarians and vegans the easiest and most pleasant ways to make sure you have sufficient sulfates are to use Epsom Salt baths regularly. The elements very readily get absorbed through your skin and enter the bloodstream rapidly. From there they find the places where they are needed and start to promote health in a variety of ways.

So why are sulfates so important?

They are what protect us from arthritis, kickstart our digestive processes by causing cascades of enzymes to start working on our food. They also help brain tissue form and are critical in the developing embryo of a baby. For example, at a point in the baby's pre-birth development sulfates are needed to build the neurones which will become the light switches in the baby's brain as they begin to grow. The neurones start connecting with one another once the infant's brain begins interacting with the outside world from the moment they are born and this is what develops a human brain.

Through a process of chemical binding it helps us detox from all kinds of contaminants, for example: drugs, heavy metals, pollution in the environment, contamination of foods we eat. This is a vital aid to our bodies as an overloaded body full of toxins becomes sluggish and inefficient in many of the processes needed to keep you healthy. A regular detox is a good idea and suggestions for how best to do that are covered in the Health section of this eBook.

Why do we need Epsom Salt now more than ever?

This brings us to a relevant fact about modern diets. This is not a problem our man, Henry in Epsom would have encountered, as he did not eat a Standard Western diet with many highly processed foods. Think refined flour, sugar, margarine and dairy which tend to be part of our everyday intake. All of these work against the absorption and processing of magnesium and sulfates and leave us in a depleted state. We also tend not to eat sufficient green vegetables, plenty of nuts and oily seeds like flax to make up for what we are not able to access. This means that it can be helpful to take Magnesium supplements to boost our body levels of this vital element and to begin taking regular (3 times/week) Epsom Salt baths so that both magnesium and sulfate can be soaked into the body. The next section will show you how.

Chapter 2

Epsom Salt Baths and Your Health

With the history of 'taking the waters' which was an annual practice for many of the gentry in Regency England the idea of creating your own 'spa' in your home has become standard for us today. However there is a long history of the practice of bathing as a health promoter. Not only England had Spa Towns, but on the Continent, where places like Baden-Baden in Germany's Black Forest welcomed European royalty to its glorious spa buildings, the idea of self-care through using natural remedies influenced a very strong tradition of alternative health in Europe too.

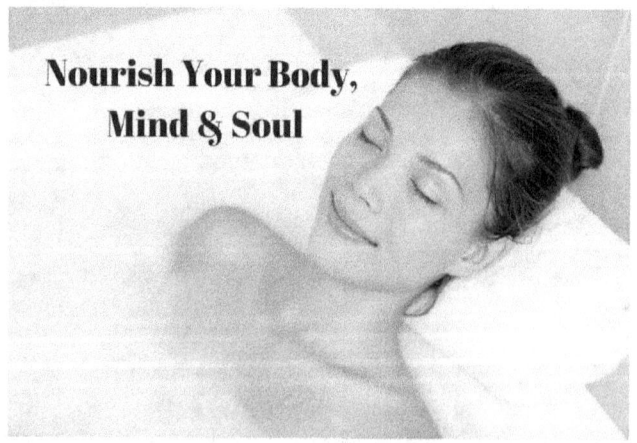

So now it is time to go to your bathroom and look at it with fresh eyes. Think about what the spas of yesteryear had that made them so good at supporting good health and curing some ills that were not responsive to other forms of medicine.

For this we need to go back in our time machine even further into the past and visit the baths in Roman and Greek times when these civilizations were at their height.

The History of Spas and Health Care

Bathing was an incredibly important activity in Roman times and most towns had hundreds of bathing houses. The wealthy had private baths and that is the trend we have carried on in our modern homes. However the rich Romans would have had several bathing rooms, each with a different type of cleansing experience such as steaming, cold water baths or warm water baths. Do you see already how you might use your bathroom creatively to make different experiences for yourself?

Even earlier in history the Greeks started the practice of having small bathing containers for foot care and hand care. Gradually the 'containers' became larger and began holding a whole body, similar to the baths we know. The Romans however carried this even further and built baths which became large enough for many bathers to share. The whole trip to the local baths became a social event as well as a practical one for washing off the dust and keeping one's body clean. Business deals, liaisons and friendships were conducted in these public Baths and the very small cost of using the services put the baths within reach of everyone.

From entering the baths the person started with the cold water tank and progressed through tepid baths to the hottest water, then returned via a tepid bath again and there began the process of massage with oils, scraping of the skin to clean and rejuvenate it. During this they paid close attention to the condition of their bodies as they took their time to relax and regain not only a clean state of body – but also a settling and calming of their minds. In some of the best public baths they then moved on to a dry room where they could rest and relax some more before being ready to re-enter their lives.

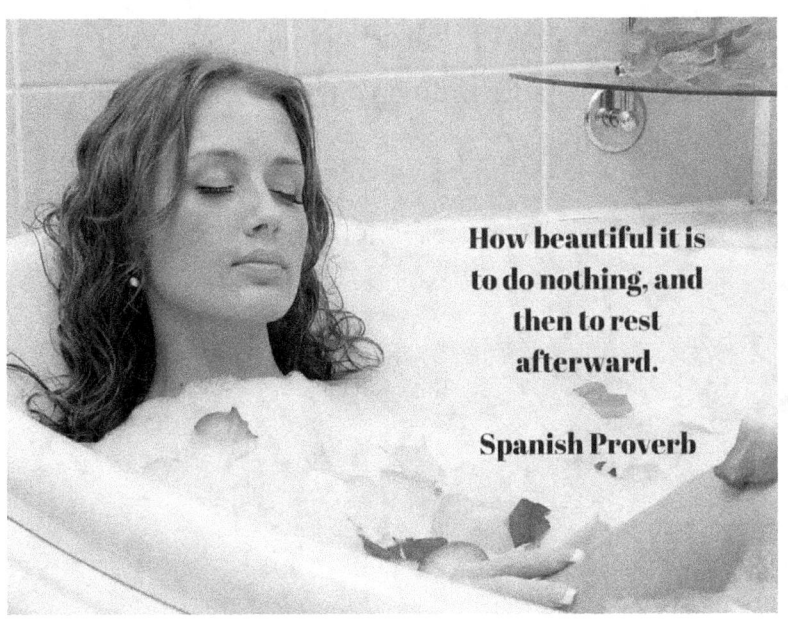

> How beautiful it is to do nothing, and then to rest afterward.
>
> **Spanish Proverb**

To try at home. Give yourself the time you need to make bathing and soaking an integral and necessary part of your health routine. Make it as important to you as brushing your teeth and combing your hair. Perhaps in today's world we can't do this every day, unlike the Romans, but we could have an evening a week, or a weekend morning or afternoon to devote to ourselves. Take the time to soak and adjust the temperature of the water as you lie there. Use Epsom Salt and a variety of essential oils to soak in through your skin as you lie and drift. Do not use soap as this makes the salts less effective. As the water drains use moisturizers and salves to dress any areas where you have bruises or very dry skin, then wrap yourself in a warmed fluffy towel or dressing gown and lie quietly on the bed as you dry off. This gives the salts, oils and salves the best chance to sink deeply into your tissues, easing aches and pains and healing your system.

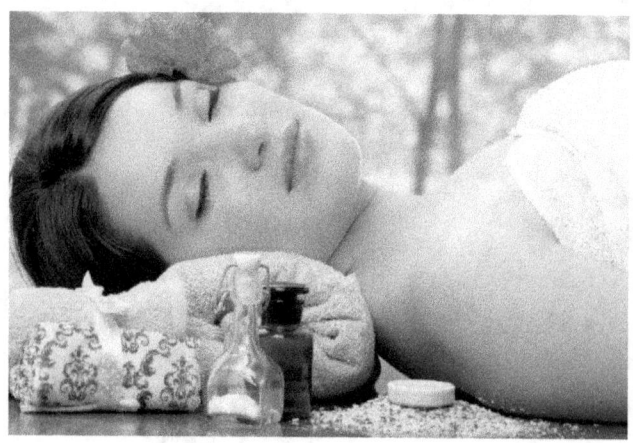

This is one of the most de-stressing ways to spend an hour (or more). If you make it a routine and insist that you have your 'me time' families grow to respect your privacy and in the end may well start to copy you!

The Romans were exceptionally civilized people and they decorated their bathing rooms in beautiful ceramics, and designs which brought the sea to mind, such as sculptures of dolphins and sea creatures. They also had the bathing areas open to the gardens and this allowed bathers to soak their senses in greenery, flowers, birdsong and gentle breezes as well as soaking up the water and minerals. All in all the

Romans understood the importance of making a gorgeous sensuous experience of their ablutions and this influenced them positively at body, mind and spirit levels.

To try at home: bring plants into your bathroom. Take the trouble to bring a beautiful flower blossom into the bathroom and put it where you can quietly rest your gaze on it, noticing it's symmetry, its energy, color, scent … This is a way to be mindful and bring in a simple meditative practice to help relieve your stress and allow your nervous system to move into 'relaxation mode' rather than the typical 'action' mode.

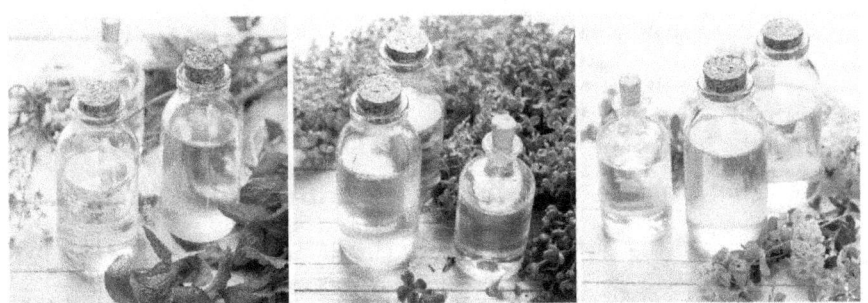

When you are buying Epsom Salt to begin your everyday use of its amazing properties be aware that there are 3 types of Epsom Salt

Don't worry, it is unlikely that you will buy the wrong type as they tend to be sold in very different stores or departments depending on the purpose you have for it.

1. Food grade or USP Grade (United States Pharmaceutical Grade) which is quality controlled and therefore pure. These are the Epsom Salt that you will find in the personal care range of products and in the grocery store. Here it will be sold in small quantities of plus/minus 500g and is likely to cost less than a bottle of shampoo.
2. Technical Grade which is for Agricultural use and is therefore a less tested and quality controlled product. Also known as Industrial Grade and can be used in mass amounts for fertilizing. In fact it will be sold in large bags for this purpose.
3. Asian Epsom Salt which is made abroad in China or Asia and is not regulated to the same extent as those made in America or Europe. This certainly makes them cheaper but they may well have impurities in them such as heavy metals and are best avoided.

Chapter 3
Health Tips for Epsom Salts

If you think about the body and all the extraordinary processes that are involved in being alive and being healthy we can see just what an awe-inspiring thing the body really is. We can also start to understand just how many things can go wrong if its systems get out of balance. This is why it is so important to have regular health care habits so that we service our bodies in the same way we service our cars. Preventive action is always easier and more efficient than a knee-jerk response to something going wrong.

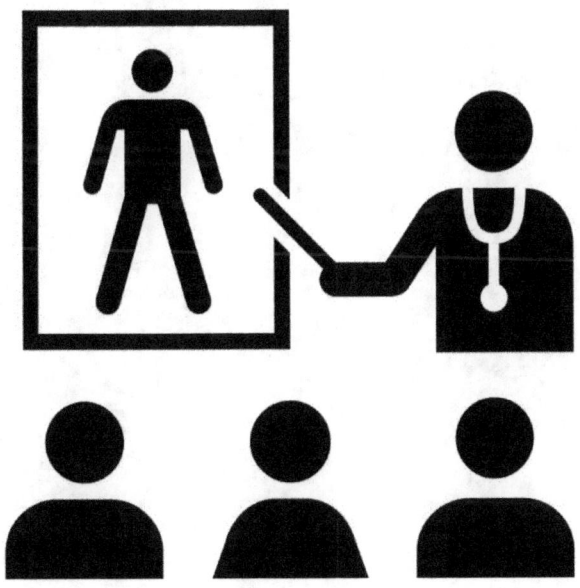

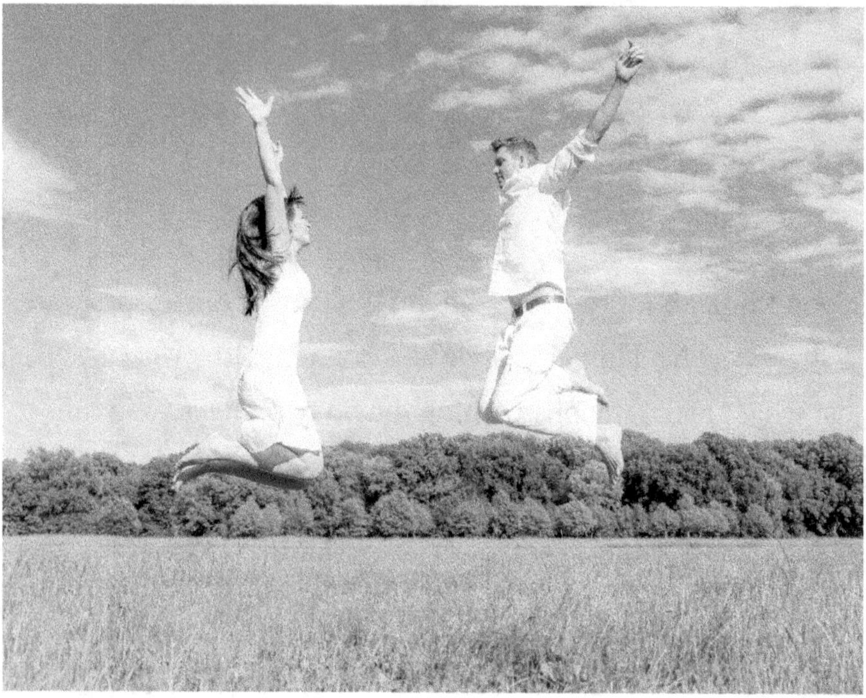

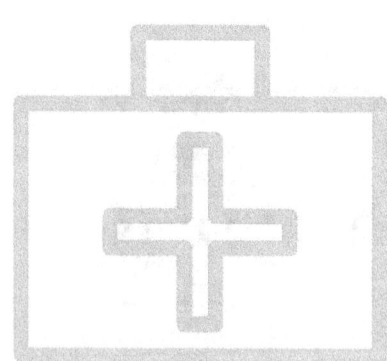

There are 10 systems in the body:

1. Cardiovascular
2. Nervous
3. Endocrine
4. Skin
5. Digestive
6. Reproductive
7. Skeletal
8. Muscular
9. Respiratory
10. Urinary

Of course, all these systems work together and support one another to make the whole body, mind and spirit healthy. However, what more than half of them have in common is that magnesium is an essential element in their efficient working. Thus directly, or indirectly, magnesium influences everything!

Sulfates too are indispensable as they work at a different level influencing the functioning of enzymes, particularly those in the stomach and digestive system, the production of amino acids which are building blocks for protein in our bodies (muscle) and forming antioxidants which help to reduce inflammation and infection.

Understanding the Body's Need for Epsom Salt and other minerals

Nervous system

Benefits: Stress reduction, sleep improvement, relief from migraine and tension headaches.

This is where magnesium eases stress and promotes deep relaxation. Low levels of magnesium lead to the body producing less serotonin. As one of the neurotransmitters responsible for our 'feel good' states we can end up low and depressed without enough of this biochemical. If you are taking enough through the regular use of Epsom Salt your appetite will be stable, your sleep will be regular and many people report a dropping off in the frequency of migraine headaches.

Muscular system

Benefits: Relieves aches and muscle cramps.

Typical aches and pains for many people are caused by arthritis and osteoporosis which has been associated with calcium deficiency. However, without magnesium calcium cannot be absorbed properly and that can lead to one of the two types of arthritis (osteo or rheumatoid). It doesn't help to take calcium tablets alone as calcium can then collect in the tissues but still not be absorbed properly into the bloodstream and bones. Make sure that if you are taking a supplement it contains both elements. Even taking magnesium tablets alone will improve calcium take up in the body – and that might be all you need.

Cardiovascular system

<u>Benefits: Heart protection and circulation improvement</u>

Eases the heart and helps to prevent hardening of the arteries and stops blood clots forming. The magnesium in Epsom Salt is a powerful heart protector. Given how prevalent heart disease is with its high blood pressure, raised cholesterol levels and disturbed eating patterns, symptoms which all point to the start of Syndrome X (metabolic syndrome) it makes sense to take preventive action early on. Have a look at your family history and if there are signs of heart disease running in the family – hypertension, heart attacks or strokes – get into the habit of taking those baths and adding in Epsom Salt to your routine right now. As a side benefit the Salt helps to improve your circulation so that if you add in some regular exercise to your routine too you are giving yourself an even better chance of protection.

Digestive System

<u>Constipation relief, optimum use of nutrients in food</u>

Relieves constipation and works with the digestive system to make it more efficient at absorbing nutrients from food. Because the Epsom Salt with its dosage of hydrated magnesium and sulfate helps fluid to be absorbed into the digestive tract, food waste becomes moist and it is able to pass more easily, and painlessly, along the elimination organs. It also helps to tone the cells and smooth muscle of the digestive system which mends leaky gut syndrome and helps food matter pass quickly through the different stages of digestion allowing the body to absorb the nutrients its needs rapidly.

However the ways in which Epsom Salt can help the digestive system don't stop there. The other great benefit of the Salt is that it can reduce inflammation. More people are understanding now just how inflamed our bodies can become. Mostly this is to do with our diets which stack up refined produce and keep us eating foods which bring the body tissues into a state of acidity. The acidity works on joints, muscle and at cellular levels throughout the body reducing their efficiency and seriously jeopardizing health long term. We need to make the body more alkaline to balance all that acidity and reduce the inflammation. We can do this by having a diet far heavier in leafy greens and stopping taking sugar, refined white flour and processed meats as part of our daily consumption.

The benefits of a better-balanced Ph in your body are many:

* you will recuperate more quickly from any disease,

* cuts will heal quickly and cleanly,

* bruises will fade rapidly

* bacterial infections and viral attacks will be less severe or not even start

* inflammation from sunburn will be reduced So don't forget to pack a box of Epsom Salt when you go on holiday. Make up a spray which you spritz on your exposed skin regularly, especially after a period in direct sunlight.)

* swollen areas will be reduced in size, since much of that swelling is caused by the body trying to lessen the amount of inflammation internally.

Endocrine System

<u>Benefits: Reduces blood sugar</u>

The endocrine system is where you secrete and balance hormones and where your needs for adrenalin, insulin, oestrogen, testosterone and other vital biochemicals are managed. As you can imagine this system is essential to feeling well and balanced. One of the most important jobs the magnesium within the Epsom Salt has is to make insulin more effective in the body. It helps the insulin in your body to be an effective blood sugar reducer.

Having the right amount of magnesium daily can reduce your blood sugar by more than 30%. The good news is that you can get a daily dose through soaking in an Epsom Salt bath as the magnesium is absorbed so readily through the skin., What an excellent excuse for that nightly 'dialling down for sleep' soak in the bath.

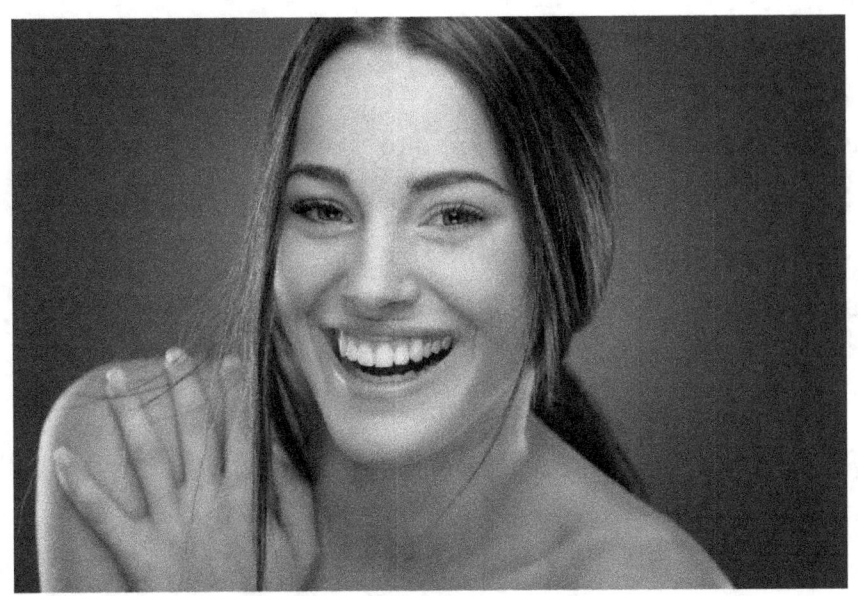

Skin, nails, hair system

Benefits: eliminate infections, cleanses, antibiotic action

A mammoth system used for protection of the whole body skin, nails and hair play a crucial part in looking after you. One of the biggest advantages of skin is that it is permeable, in other words elements such as magnesium, sulfates etc. can pass through the top layer of the skin. The elements then get absorbed into the blood and lymph systems and begin to circulate through the body finding the parts which need the minerals most. Think about how we get our daily dose of Vitamin D – straight from sunlight through our skin and into our body. This means we can use our skin to nourish ourselves at a very deep level, very easily.

You can develop some diseases of this protective layer such as a fungus which can invade the nail bed, athlete's foot which can affect the skin on the feet and toes or acne where the pores become deeply infected. All of these conditions can be treated through absorbing Epsom Salt. Use a foot bath if you are short of time or an Epsom Salt compress for your face.

Urinary System

Benefits: Detoxifies the whole body.

The urinary system is designed to carry toxins out of the body and to continually give us the equivalent of an internal wash. Some of the more dangerous things that we absorb from the food we eat, the water we drink and the air we breathe are the so-called 'heavy metals'. The ones we are most aware of are cadmium, mercury, lead and arsenic. Remember the old stories about the dandies and ladies in Elizabethan times dying from lead poisoning because they used a lead based whitening powder on their faces! Well, we don't use that now but we still have many objects in our environment that leak lead and the other metals which we end up absorbing in roundabout ways. One of the problems with heavy metals is that they tend to sink into the tissues and not be flushed out through any other system. Using Epsom Salt the heavy metals then have something else to bind with and the magnesium sulfate with its 'passenger' of heavy metal is able to be swept through the system and away. This leaves the body tissues far healthier and is an excellent way to detox.

To try at Home

Instructions for Salt Baths

All of these systems can be accessed by using Epsom salts in a bath. It is advised that this is done 3 times/week for the best benefits.

The amount of Epsom Salt to be used is at least 2 full cups of the Salt. It depends of course on how full you like your bath to be and if you are one of those people who like to float in their bath then up to 500g of Epsom Salt would work well to a tub of water.

Twelve to twenty minutes is the average amount of time to stay in the water to allow the absorption of the elements. Remember that you can also gradually increase, then decrease the temperature of the water to echo the Roman Bathing techniques. Even better is then to lie down for up to an hour while your body dries and heals as Nature intended.

If you are using a footbath as a shorter, quicker pick me up, use half a cup of Epsom Salt and let your feet soak for ten minutes before wrapping them up in a warm towel and lying down for a few more minutes.

Instructions for Epsom Salt Drinks

Bathing, although a sensuous and gorgeous way to support good health, is not the only way to obtain the benefits of Epsom Salt. Going back to our history lesson again the whole movement began with people drinking the waters. In fact in Epsom itself, at its height, visitors were drinking up to sixteen pints/day! That is quite a shock to the system. Not advised today, but the following recipes will help you with your detoxing regime and give gentle support to your liver and excretory organs.

Gentle Detox with Epsom Salt

There are some important facts to know about before you begin any detox routine. These are especially important to remember when using Epsom Salt as they are so powerful and beneficial you need to understand how to best help your body.

1. It takes two days to detox so plan to do this over a weekend or during a holiday.
2. Before you begin buy in:
- A grapefruit (people on cardiac management medication need to check if grapefruit is safe to mix with the medicine you are taking). If you are in any doubt rather use an orange or half a teaspoon of baking soda in the mix.
- Extra virgin olive oil.
- Plenty of fresh filtered water to drink throughout the regime.
3. Magazines or books/videos/CD's you have been planning to get to 'sometime'.
4. Don't plan any activity during the two days – just think of them as 'Totally Me Time' and enjoy the rest.
5. The day you plan to start have a no-fat breakfast and lunch. This would be toast and honey or fruit puree, a bowl of vegetables and rice or a cereal grain like quinoa. This is done to place no extra stress on your liver.
6. Stop drinking or eating by 2 pm on your first day.

Detox Regime.

Mix together:

- 4 tablespoons Epsom Salt
- 3 cups filtered water

Instructions:

1. Store in fridge.
2. Drink your first three-quarters of a cup of Epsom Salt mix around 6 pm on Day 1. If the slightly 'soapy' taste is unpleasant for you add a squirt of lemon juice or orange juice to adjust it to suit you.
3. Drink your second three-quarters of a cup of the mixture at 8 pm. Keep resting.
4. Make up a cup of olive oil (half a cup) and grapefruit juice half a cup (or alternative) and mix together thoroughly. Let stand.
5. At 10 pm drink the oil mixture. You can flavor this if you find it hard to swallow – but gulping it down quickly to get it finished works too!
6. Rest quietly for the remainder of the night.
7. In the morning when you wake up take the next three-quarters of a cup of Epsom Salt mix.
8. Go back to bed and rest again for two hours.
9. Around 10 am take the last cup of Epsom Salt mix.

10. Rest again for 2 hours and then drink some fruit juice of your choice.
11. After half an hour you can have some lovely slices of cut up fruit such as apples, bananas, paw paw, mango.....
12. In another half hour a light meal of salad/vegetables and fish/chicken.

Dinner can be whatever you would normally have.

Do not take yourself far from the bathroom as you are likely to have a short spell of diarrhea at this point. Keep taking it easy although you can now be a bit more active since you have been eating.

Epsom Salts as a Laxative

If you don't want to go through the Detox regime but you have been suffering from some constipation, Epsom Salt helps in this case too.

Recipe:

1. Mix together 2 teaspoons of Epsom Salt in one cup of filtered water.
2. Stir it well and add some lemon juice or a teaspoon of lemon/orange or cranberry juice if you'd like to make it more palatable.

3. Drink this cupful two times/day leaving at least 4 hours between each dose.
4. As with the detox make sure you stay close to the bathroom as it can start working anytime between half an hour to six hours after drinking depending on your age, weight and type of metabolism.

Keep drinking plenty of water to keep your digestive track moist and your cells well hydrated. If it is more convenient for you - you can make up a jug of the Laxative mix by tripling the amounts above and keep it refrigerated so that you can just pour your twice daily dose from the jug at the right times. Remember to stir well each time as sometimes the Epsom Salt takes a while to dissolve.

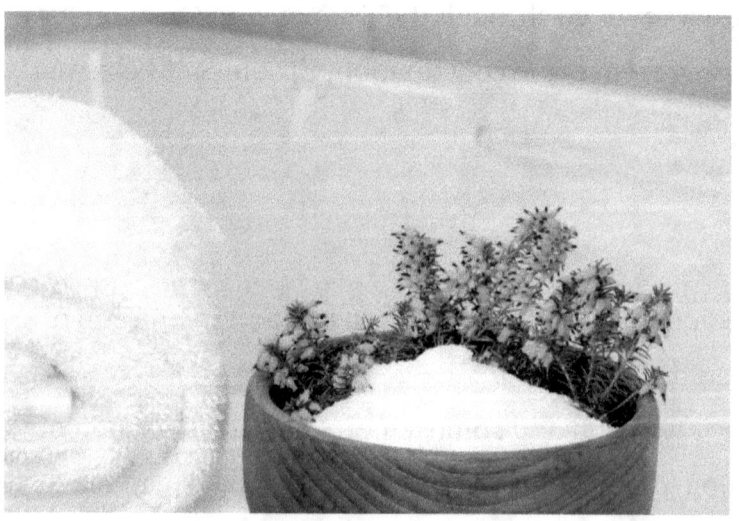

Chapter 4
First Aid and Epsom Salt

Our Epsom Salt is such a good all-rounder that it is also an idea to keep some in a bottle in your first aid kit. The everyday cuts, bruises, stings and splinters can all be healed with the help of Epsom Salt.

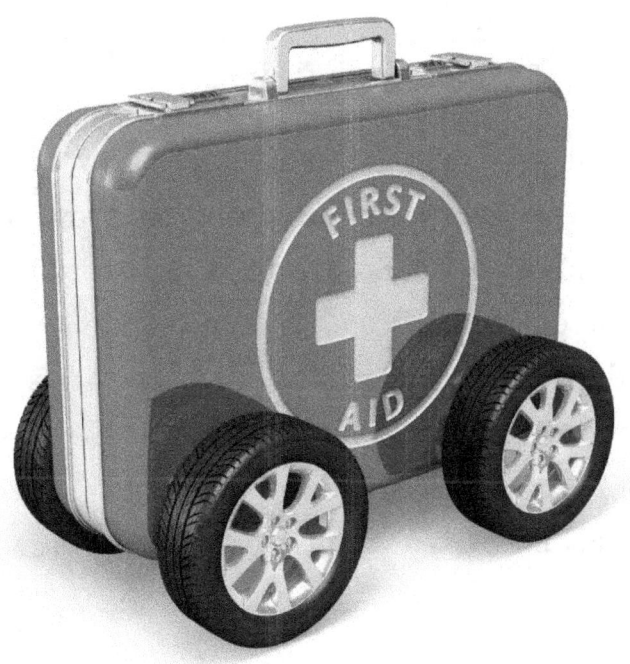

Bug bites and bee sting

Two and a half tablespoons of Epsom Salt well mixed into a cup of cold water make an excellent concentrated solution for tackling bites and stings. Pour some of the solution on a cotton pad or facecloth and keep applying to the site of the bite or sting until the redness and discomfort have died down. Remember that if you have trouble breathing after a sting you may be allergic and you need to see a doctor/hospital immediately.

Hangover

A bit of over-indulgence can leave you feeling sluggish and lethargic. These are signs of some toxicity in your body and just a quarter of a teaspoon of Epsom Salt in half a cup of warm water will settle things down. It's important to remember to drink plenty of fresh filtered water with this remedy so that you really flush your system out and keep hydrated. For better results, add some lemon or grapefruit juice. Also, avoid caffeine as it will make you even more dehydrated.

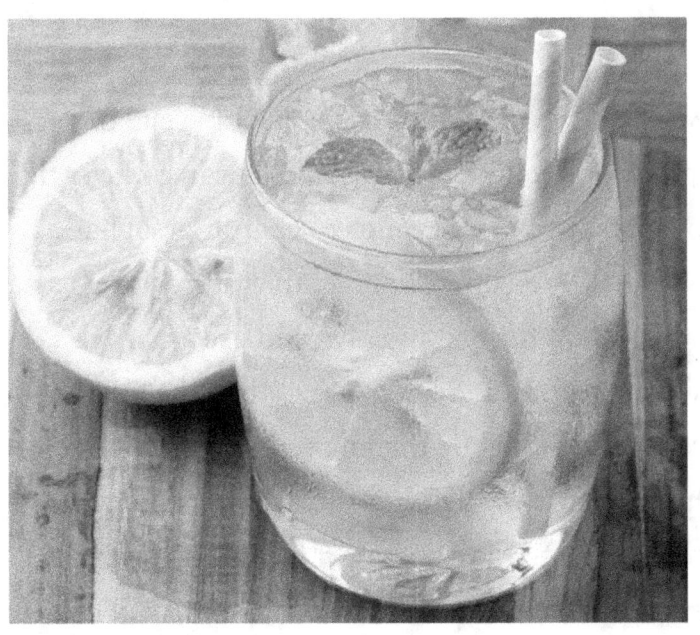

Splinter and Bruise Help

Similar to the string and bite remedy Epsom Salt can be used to reduce the swelling, inflammation and discoloration of bruises or splinters. Making a solution of two tablespoons of Epsom Salt and a cup of cold water works as an effective compress when a cloth pad is soaked in it and applied to the affected site. Keep the wet cloth on the area until it begins to warm up with the heat of your skin, then squeeze out and soak again in the solution. Apply again and keep doing this for five or six applications. This helps to combat any infection as well as the remaining inflammation.

Eye wash

Sometimes we can develop a painful stye on our eyelid or contract conjunctivitis (pink eye). Epsom Salt can come to the rescue here by making up a very mild concentration of half teaspoon Epsom Salt to a cup of blood temperature water (just tepid). Mix well so that the Salt dissolve and use as an eye bath or as a warm compress. Soak a facecloth in the weak solution and squeeze out lightly then place over the infected eye. Allow the cloth to cool slightly then keep refreshing the cloth in the solution until the discomfort in your eye lessens slightly. Keep repeating every couple of hours until you can see the improvement in the tissue.

Warts

Warts can make an unpleasant appearance on your skin and a quick and easy way to turn to natural remedies to help yourself is to mix together 1 tablespoon Epsom Salt with 4 tablespoons Apple Cider Vinegar. Keep this in the fridge and use cotton swabs to dab some onto the warts 3 – 5 times/day. Just allow the liquid to dry off itself each time which will leave a coat of solution on the warts in between treatments. Keep this up for 5 days and see how it helps them to heal.

As well as keeping a wound from a splinter free from infection Epsom Salt can also contribute to extracting the splinter itself using the power it has to draw water out of tissue. The change in osmotic pressure will help the splinter move to the surface of its own accord. Achieve this by soaking the place where the splinter is lodged in a mix of 2 tablespoons of Epsom Salt to one cup of water.

Epilepsy and MS

In the Health section we paid a lot of attention to Epsom Salt as a relaxant and as something that promotes sound sleep and stress relief. For those of you who have Multiple Sclerosis, Epilepsy, ME or asthma which can be triggered by stress it is a good idea to support yourself as much as possible by having a daily warm Epsom Health bath. The doses of Magnesium will help you sleep better and the practice of daily relaxation – especially if you enhance it through mediation or just having a quiet time in the bath – will mean that your nervous system will learn to stay in the Relaxation mode of the parasympathetic system longer each day. This will reduce the excitation of the sympathetic nervous system and make less work for your body.

Chapter 5

Epsom Salt and Beauty

We now have a thorough understanding of the many ways in which Epsom Salt with its unique combination of magnesium and sulfate helps us to maintain our natural well-being, and correct our health issues before they get too established. Remember prevention is always better than cure. Though cure is a real bonus too!

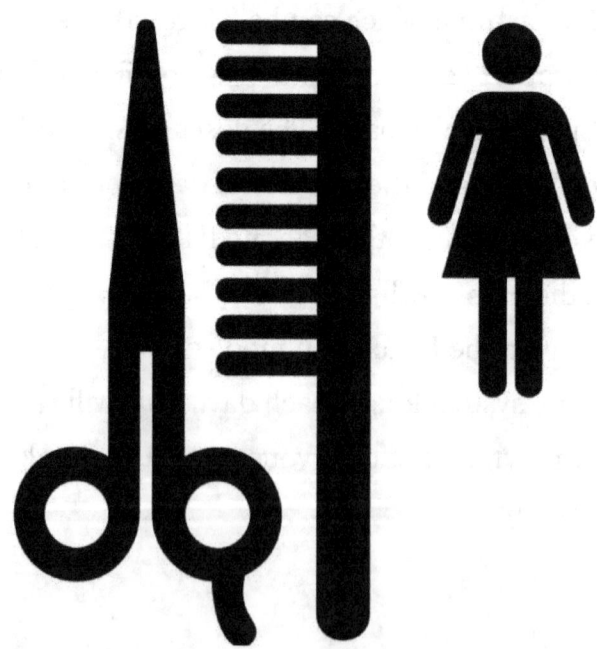

Health is bound up with Beauty and as you might expect there are many ways Epsom salts can be used to boost your beauty, and benefit your health too. In this section we will look at the best methods for using Epsom Salt as beauty aids and highlight the specific benefits each one brings.

Before we start on this section it is a good idea to check out your bathroom and kitchen cupboards for other natural products you have which can be combined with Epsom salts to make wonderful new mixtures to pamper yourself at every level.

Moisturising cream: your favourite whatever it is:

- Essential oils – particularly peppermint, eucalyptus, lavender, thyme
- Bentonite clay
- Petroleum jelly
- Coffee grounds
- Sesame oil - extra virgin if possible
- Olive oil and coconut oil
- Tomato
- Aloe Vera gel
- Chamomile Tea (if you have fair hair)

- Black Tea (if you have dark hair)
- Favorite hair conditioner

Skin:

Exfoliation

Use Epsom salts as an exfoliating cream by adding in half a teaspoon of Salt to the usual amount of facial cleanser you use. Stir them together and apply to your face then rinse off with cool water. The cool water will act as a toner for your skin and the Epsom Salt will help to lift off the top layer of skin cells which are ready to come off as the new, fresh skin emerges below.

Anti-aging

Anti-aging properties in Epsom Salt from the hydrated magnesium and sulfate help to lessen the aging effect of oxidation and environmental pollution. Make this a great way to make your own facial deep cleanse and anti-wrinkle cream too. Just leave the facial cleanser and Epsom Salt mix you made above on your face for ten minutes or more before you wipe it off with the cool damp cloth.

Body cleansing

Shower Sock

For those hit and run moments when a bath would be nice but a shower is more practical just grab a couple of handfuls of Epsom Salt and rub them over your body. Let the shower sluice away the grains of salt and leave your skin smooth and soft.

If you have an old white sock you can fill it with Epsom Salt and tie the top with a pretty piece of ribbon to secure the salt. Keep this in your shower and use it as a body wipe to help detox, exfoliate and smooth your body. Once the salt has dissolved the sock can be refilled again.

Milk Baths

Epsom Salt is so good for bathing in for health reasons that it makes sense to incorporate them into your routine beauty bathing too. Milk baths are popular because they moisturize your skin and add a bit of a luxury to bathtime. Before you get into the bath:

1. Add together half a cup of powdered milk (personally I love almond milk as it smells wonderful) and half a cup of Epsom Salt.
2. Drop in three drops of any essential oil of your choice.

3. Rose essential oil is a particularly sweet oil to use for this – but if you have a favourite such as ylang-ylang use that.
4. The oil is just to make the occasion into a deluxe experience!
5. Add a splash of water. Just enough to make a paste so be sure to add a tablespoon at a time so you can control the consistency.
6. Once your paste is made, rub it onto the dry skin areas on your body.
7. Favourite areas are elbows and feet but often dry scaly patches can start anywhere if you have been out in the sun.
8. Give yourself a minute or two for the paste to harden on your skin then pop into the bath and soak.
9. If there is any extra paste in the bowl tip it into the bath too.

Give yourself at least 20 minutes of luxuriating time and then wipe off any remaining paste with the facecloth.

Get out of the bath and enjoy the sensation of softness and perfume surrounding you.

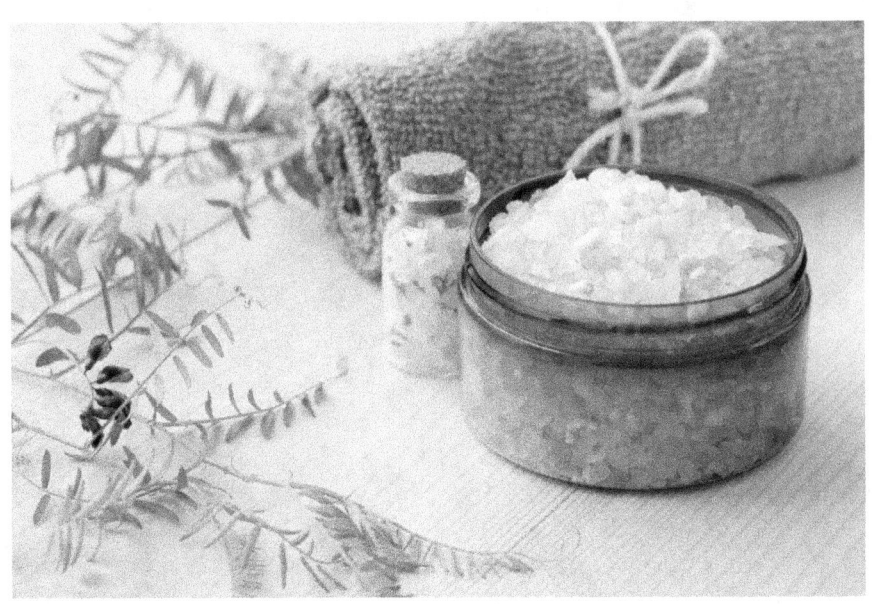

Epsom Salt Bath Bombs

Before you start, assemble the following ingredients:

Dry Ingredients

- 1 cup Baking Soda
- Half cup Citric acid powder
- Half cup Epsom Salt

Wet ingredients

- 2 teaspoons Olive oil
- 2 teaspoons Witch Hazel

- 1 teaspoon Vanilla essence
- Essential oil of your choice such as citrus, bergamot ...
- Dried herb of your choice such as ginger powder
- Silicon baking moulds or muffin pans.
- Bowl to mix in
- Wooden spoon

Instructions:

1. Mix together the dry ingredients and put aside.
2. Mix together the wet ingredients and stir them well.
3. Quickly add the dry and the wet ingredients together and mix well using a spoon or your hands.
4. The mixture should stick together like a pastry dough with no crumbling.
5. Add a little water or more witch hazel if it is still a bit dry.
6. Then quickly roll into balls and push into the silicon molds or greased muffin pans. Press each one in firmly and cover.
7. Leave to dry and if you peep under the cover from time to time and notice that they are expanding this is right.
8. Just gently push them down again to stop them from expanding too much.

9. After they are dry (a day or two) put them in an airtight container and store.

These bombs last up to a year and are great presents too.

Masks and Moisturizing

Getting rid of acne – and removing blackheads – can be done by adding a teaspoon of Epsom salts to 3 drops of iodine and mixing into a half cup of hot water. Using a cotton swab wipe over the infected or blocked pores. Leave for a couple of minutes then again sluice off with lukewarm water.

For chronic acne another home remedy using Epson Salt is to whip up one egg white until it forms stiff peaks, add in a teaspoon of aloe vera, a teaspoon of Epsom Salt, a mashed up ripe tomato and a half teaspoon of Vit B5 powder then drip in one or two drops of an essential oil of your choice. Thyme or Lavender are both good as they are antibiotic and soothing. Smooth into face or areas where acne is severe and wait for a quarter of an hour before rinsing off. Doing this regularly can have a wonderful effect on the infected areas.

Petroleum Jelly (a quarter of a cup) added to two cups of Epsom Salt makes another excellent mask and a deep penetrating moisturizer. Great for the hardened skin on the soles of your feet or calluses on your hands. Also you can use this as a gentle gloss for your lips when they become chapped by winter wind and cold.

Bentonite clay is another excellent companion for Epsom Salt when you want to make a mask. Mixed together they can be used for facial masks or body masks.

For a body mask use:

- Half a cup of Bentonite Clay powder (Ebay is a good source)
- Half a cup Epsom Salt
- A drop of the essential oil of your choice.

Instructions:

1. Pour the Epsom Salt into the bath water and add the drop of essential oil.
2. Put a small amount of water in the cup with the Clay and make up a stiff paste.

3. Mix well using a wooden spoon (not metal) so that the lumps work themselves out.
4. Smear the paste on your body and give yourself another 5 minutes of air drying the paste before climbing into the Epsom Salt and essential oil bath.
5. Soak for at least 20 minutes.
6. Use the facecloth for removing any last bits of clay as you get out of the bath.
7. As you will know from the Health Section this is a powerful combination as the Bentonite Clay works to pull out toxins from the body and the Epsom Salt also detoxifies the body and gently releases the sulfate and magnesium to be absorbed through the skin.
8. Bear in mind that the warmer you have the water the stronger the detox will be and this means that you will gain the most benefit by resting and relaxing on the bed afterwards.

Hair Care

<u>Make a hairspray</u>

Tired of having your eyes water and sneezing your head off after a spray of bought 'hair product'? Making your own with Epsom Salt is a great, and very economical, option.

- 3 tablespoons Epsom salt

- Half a teaspoon pink sea salt or Himalayan Salt
- 1 teaspoon Aloe Vera gel
- 2 drops of essential oil, choosing one of your favourite scents
- 1 cup of hot tea as the base. Use Chamomile for light hair and Black, everyday tea for dark hair.
- I spray bottle which can be bought from many chemists

Instructions:

1. Add all ingredients to the bottle and shake well until the Salts are dissolved.
2. Store this in your fridge between uses and it will last up to four months.

<u>Remove hairspray</u>

On the other hand sometimes you can have a build up of hair spray on your hair which makes it looks dull. In this case you can use your Epsom Salt again to come to the rescue.

- 2 litres water
- Half cup lemon juice
- Half cup Epsom Salt.

Instructions:

1. Mix together and leave overnight.
2. The next day pour the mixture on your dry hair before washing it.
3. Wrap an old towel around your head and do something else for 20 minutes.
4. After this wash your hair as normal and enjoy how soft, refreshed and shiny it has become.

Volumize hair

There are some days when your hair just seems to be lank. Or maybe you have long fine hair that lies in smooth straight sheets, but you want some volume in it when you go out. Epsom Salt steps into the breach again:

Take:

- Half a cup of your best deep hair conditioner
- Half a cup of Epsom Salt

Instructions:

1. Stir these together and gently warm in a pan.
2. Then take the warmed mixture and work it into your dry hair.

3. Using an old towel wrap this around your treated hair and wait for twenty minutes. Rinse your hair thoroughly and style as usual.

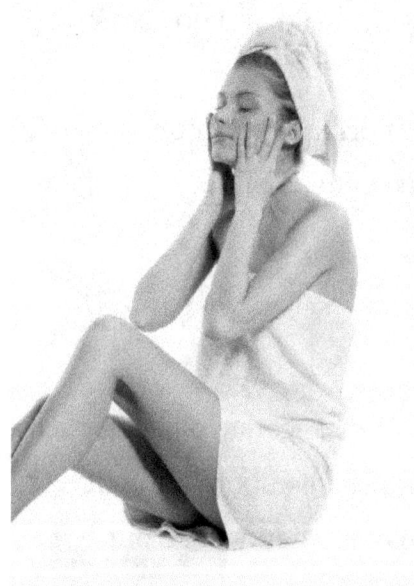

Hair Protection

If you are having some pampering time at your local beauty spa or swimming baths Epsom Salt can protect your hair when it is in the harsher environment of the steam room, sauna or chlorinated pool. Using the same recipe as above put the warmed and combined mixture in a jar and take it to the Spa. Enjoy a swim then when you come out of the pool coat your hair with the mixture and pull on a hair turban or wrap a towel around your head and then go into the steam or heat rooms.

Twenty minutes or more to let the Salt do its magic and then rinse off in the shower. Comb through and style.

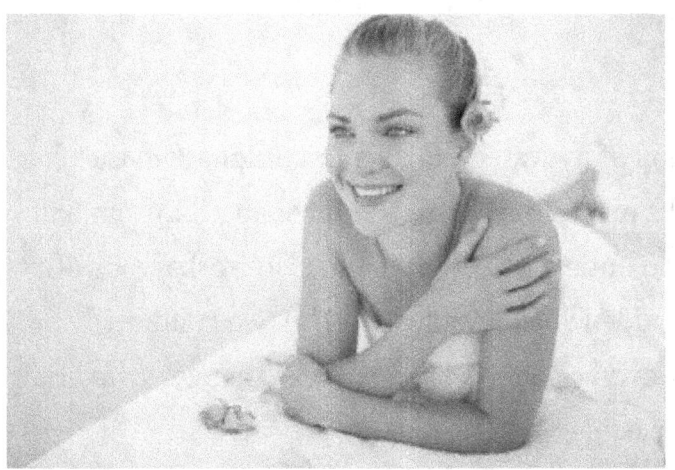

It also works well if you enjoy all the spa treatment rooms and then wash your hair, apply the mix, wrap your towel around your head and go through to the resting lounge. A browse through a magazine will take up about twenty minutes and then a quick rinse off in the shower again before you style your hair and get dressed. It is particularly useful if you use a hair dryer for styling your hair which can encourage split ends. The Epsom Salt mix strengthens your hair beautifully.

Chapter 6: Epsom Salt in Your Home

Household Uses of Epsom Salt

The introduction of hydrated Magnesium Sulphate to the household tasks makes life easier – and cheaper. Epsom Salt is a cleanser and antiseptic solution and also works well with Hydrogen Peroxide which is a bleach. The two combined make for a powerful cleaner for many areas that get grimy but are difficult to clean.

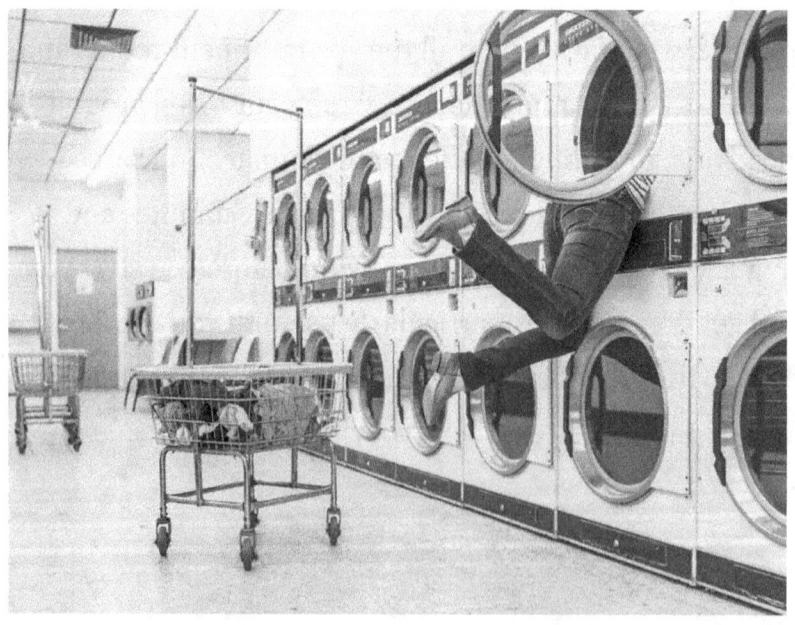

Bathroom

Wonderful for tiles and the grouting in between them. Use a toothbrush to work it in, leave for five minutes then sluice off. Polish with a clean dry cloth. Use I cup Epsom Salt to 1 cup dishwashing liquid and mix together well.

Kitchen

Using the same mix as above use around taps where an accumulation of limescale can form. Toothbrush helps to work the mix in and also acts as a slight abrasive on the lime scale, roughening it so the Epsom Salt can work into a bigger surface.

Mix half cup Epsom Salt with a quarter cup of baby oil. Add a couple of drops of a favorite essential oil too. Mix well by shaking in a jar or old shampoo bottle. Use as a hand wash to both clean and moisturize hands after working at the sink.

That hardened crust of burnt food in your pans and dishes will come right off with the help of a quarter of a tablespoon of Epsom salt and mix with the warm water you run in to soften the crust. Leave it to soak and do its work before scrubbing with a scourer and rinsing off. The crust will come off easily with this method.

Scullery/Laundry

Fill up your washing machine with hot water and throw in 3 cups of Epsom salt. Set the machine to run the 'quick' or 'economy' wash cycle. This will help to lift the detergent build up in the metal parts of the machine and clean it thoroughly.

Garage

If you have made up a solution of Epsom Salt and water for your first aid box as we looked at in the last chapter, make a double quantity and fill up another bottle for the garage too. Unbeatable for getting batteries going again when they have 'died' overnight. Just dampen the contacts and try again. Sometimes making a paste of Epsom Salt and water and putting the paste on the contact points works well too. It all depends on what you have to hand.

Front windows

It's Christmas time and you want to make pretty patterns on your windows to recreate a visit from Jack Frost. Using a bowl add 1 cup Epsom Salt to half a cup of water and stir in 3 tablespoons of dishwasher liquid.

Use a sponge to dab on the windows. As it dries the salt creates the frosting. It can easily be wiped off with a warm damp cloth later.

Chapter 7

Epsom Salt in your Garden

We already have the emergency box of Epsom salt in the garage for help with a variety of mishaps as we saw in the earlier sections. Now we make sure we have plenty of it in the potting shed – or garage – wherever you keep your garden equipment.

Epsom Salt has so many uses in the garden – fertilizer, insecticide, rescue remedy for poorly plants... Look through the following to see where you can use this plentiful and cheap powder to make your garden grow.

Fertilizer

To help new plants which you are just introducing to the garden settle in, make sure to add two or three handfuls of Epsom salt to the earth you have dug out of the hole where you will plant them. As you settle the plant into its new home pack the salted soil around the roots and stem to nourish the plant as it grows.

Use as fertilizer to help your existing plants

It is easy to deplete the ground's stock of essential elements with over planting, or by having the misfortune to live in a place where the topsoil is poor. The natural minerals needed by growing plants, such as potassium, nitrogen and phosphorus all work more effectively if they are mixed with the hydrated Magnesium Sulphate in Epsom Salt. This is especially so if you have a lot of soaking rain which dilutes the mineral all the time. Once a week go out with a bucketful of Salts and scatter a handful on your most prized flowers, houseplants and vegetables.

Grass

On an even larger scale Epsom Salt is good for the lawn to encourage new, strong and vigorous growth. Take a gallon of water and add half a cup of Epsom Salt then spray the garden with this solution. The magnesium really helps to make the green more vivid since it supports the chlorophyll production.

Flowers and Vegetables

The Salt promotes growth in two ways as it tends to make blooms or vegetables bigger and to produce more flowers/fruit or vegetables. When you are planting new flowering plants or vegetables keep scattering in Epsom salts as you plant or sow. Then keep up a weekly feed of a handful of Salt as they begin to grow. You will soon be rewarded. The most famous Epsom Salt success was a winning Pumpkin that weighed in at just over 200Kgs. A monster!

Enhance flavor in Fruit and vegetables

Epsom salt improves the flavor as well as the size and amount of your fruit and vegetables. It is particularly effective on peppers and tomatoes but any plant in your vegetable garden will benefit. Do not be afraid to use plenty of the Salt as you fertilize in this area of your garden, they can easily take three of four times as much Epsom salt as the flower garden.

Herbicide

As well as being a fertilizer for the plants you want to nurture and grow Epsom Salt can be used as a weedkiller. Mix a litre of water with 2 tablespoons of Epsom Salt and 1 tablespoon of ordinary dishing washing liquid. Shake this up then spray it on the weeds you want to get rid of and you will find that the weeds die back but the magnesium and sulphate sink into the ground leaving the soil ready for you to plant something more suitable.

Rescue Remedy for Curling Leaves

Citrus leaves can suddenly turn very curly, as can some other bushes, and this is usually a sign of lack of magnesium and is also helped by several handfuls of Epsom Salt to get the healing underway then regular handfuls weekly thereafter. Don't forget that 'skin' has the ability to absorb nutrients too and the same goes for leaves. It is possible to add Epsom Salt to your sprayer and coat the curly leaves with the solution of 1 cup Salt to 1 liter water. Make sure the salt is well dissolved first. Preferably do both the spraying and the feeding of the soil to help the curly leaves. Water the dry Salt in well so it soaks to the roots unless you know it will rain soon.

Before you plant your seedlings or new bushes soak the roots in Epsom Salt solution of half a cup of Salt to one gallon of water. Leave overnight then plant.   Let the root ball become saturated with the Salt water.

Not only roses benefit from a weekly scattering of Epsom Salts. Rhododendron and Azaleas tend to turn yellow when the sulfate level of the soil gets too low. One tablespoon over the root area every month helps with this. Water in well.

Other plants that do well with a drenching of Epsom Salt solution when they turn yellow are ferns, cycads, bougainvillea and gardenia. With their heavy flowering these last two strip the ground of magnesium so scattering half a cupful over the ground around them can replenish the lost minerals. Large leaved plants benefit from spraying with a solution of Epsom Salt made from a tablespoon of Salt to one gallon of water.

As you move into a property and start working the garden there are often old tree stumps that have been left to rot in the ground but cling tenaciously to life with parts dead and other parts very weak. Because Epsom Salt absorbs water so well it works to drill a series of holes in the trunk and pack Epsom

Salt into them. Also scatter the Salt over any old exposed roots. As the moisture is pulled out of the old stump it will become weaker and weaker and after several applications of the Salt you can uproot the old stump and start your own new project at last.

Insecticide

Slugs hate Epsom salt! So do most plant pests, so although I wouldn't stop doing your companion planting and using other natural means of pest control, spraying with Epsom salt is another addition to the arsenal against these little pests. Slugs are different! They don't like to slide over the crystals of Magnesium Sulfate so will steer clear of the areas which are regularly dusted with Epsom salt. It doesn't kill them in the way that ordinary salt does, but it does encourage them to go elsewhere!

BONUS CHAPTER

Aromatherapy Recipes & Essential Oil Blends for Your Epsom Salt Baths

The following aromatherapy recipes can be mixed with Epsom salt to enhance your Epsom salt relaxation baths! You can also use them on your own to create your holistic oils. These are fantastic for self-massage after your Epsom salt bath experience.

EO in the recipes means= essential oil

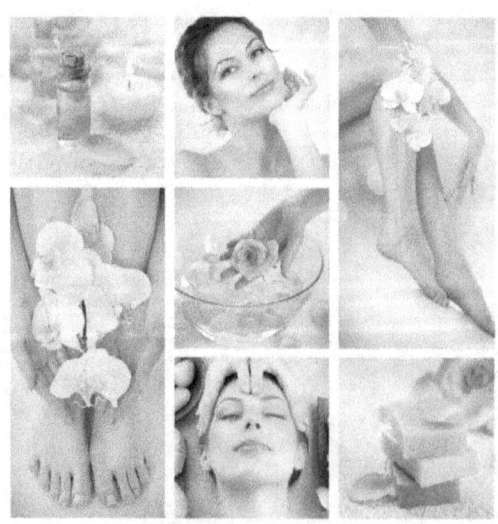

Sweet Dreams-Fight Insomnia

Blend:

- 2 tablespoons of coconut oil or olive oil (sesame oil works great too)
- 2 drops of verbena EO +
- 2 drops of lavender (or lavandin) EO +
- 2 drops of mandarin EO +

Add to your Epsom salt bath or use for self-massage.

Amazing Energy!

Sick and tired of feeling sick and tired?

Try this recipe!

Blend:

- 1 tablespoon of coconut oil
- 2 drops of Camomila Noble EO+
- 2 drops of Mandarine EO+
- 2 drops of Rosemary EO

Add to your Epsom salt bath or use for self-massage.

You can also apply via neck and head massage. It will be extremely invigorating. Moreover, head massage is a great natural hair treatment. Rosemary essential oil can help you grow strong healthy hair and prevent hair loss. It's also very energizing!

Healing Blend

Blend:

- 1 tablespoon of coconut oil or other roil (olive, sesame, almond) you like
- 2 drops of verbena EO+
- 2 drops of ylang ylang EO

Add to your Epsom salt bath or use for self-massage.

Easy Anti-Flu Mix

Blend:

- 2 tablespoons of coconut oil or other natural oil of your choice
- 2 drops of Moroccan thyme EO+
- 2 drops of eucalyptus Citriodora EO
- 2 drops of tea tree EO

Add to your Epsom salt bath or use for self-massage.

Lymphatic Help Blend

If you suffer from varicose veins, fluid retention as well as cellulite this recipe will help you rejuvenate your legs. Try to soak in an Epsom salt bath first, or add Epsom salt to your peeling. Then, prepare this aromatherapy blend for leg massage.

You can also add the following mix to your regular Epsom salt bath and take advantage of its relaxing properties, enjoy!

Blend:

- 2 tablespoons coconut oil
- 2 drops of grapefruit EO+
- 2 drops of peppermint EO+
- 2 drops of juniper EO+
- 2 drops of geranium EO

For a massage:

Massage this blend gently into your legs, start from the feet and ankles and move up so as to stimulate venous circulation.

Grapefruit, juniper and geranium work as a natural lymphatic drainage and mint gives an instant sensation of coolness and energy. Great for swollen and tired legs after a hard day at work.

Headache Remover

Blend:

- 2 tablespoons of coconut oil or other holistic oil of your choice
- 2 drops of lavandin+
- 2 drops of verbena +
- 2 drops of mint EO

Add to your Epsom salt bath or use for self-massage.

Massage instructions:

Massage forehead and temples gently and massage the neck. You can also do a scalp massage for better results, but normally a simple forehead massage (make sure you squeeze your eyebrows) will make the pain go away in less than 5 minutes.

Natural Coffee for Your Soul!

This holistic recipe will help you wake up and restore your energy levels. You can also use it for meditation, as it will help you keep centered.

Blend:

- 1 tablespoon of coconut oil
- 2 drops of citronella EO+
- 1 drop of cinnamon EO+
- 1 drops of bergamot EO+
- 1 drop of ylang ylang

Add to your Epsom salt bath or use for self-massage.

Massage instructions:

1. Massage your neck, chest, and shoulders. Head massage with oils can be extremely energizing too.
2. You will find the balance between citric scents like citronella and bergamot spiced up by floral ylang ylang fragrance and cinnamon mystery.
3. Bergamot is also a great anti-anxiety remedy as my next recipe explains.

4. Remember- no sunbathing after this massage! Citric oils are photo-toxic.

No More Anxiety!

If you feel like anxiety is knocking on your door make sure you take a few deep breaths and confide in aromatherapy and Epsom salt combo.

With this blend you can take a holistic approach and get to the root of the problem.

This is so much better than standard anti-anxiety pills that only make us sick and tired (and very often fat).

You already know that Epsom salt bath is a great source of magnesium (a mineral you need to fight stress). If you combine it with essential oils, you will give yourself an amazing mix of all natural ingredients to fight anxiety.

Blend:

- 2 tablespoons of coconut oil
- 2 drops of bergamot+
- 2 drops of verbena+
- 2 drops of basil (refrain from using this oil if you are suffering from clinical depression).

Add to your Epsom salt bath or use for self-massage.

Massage Instructions:

You can do a full body massage.

Concentrate on your feet and solar plexus.

Breathe in and out in a conscious way.

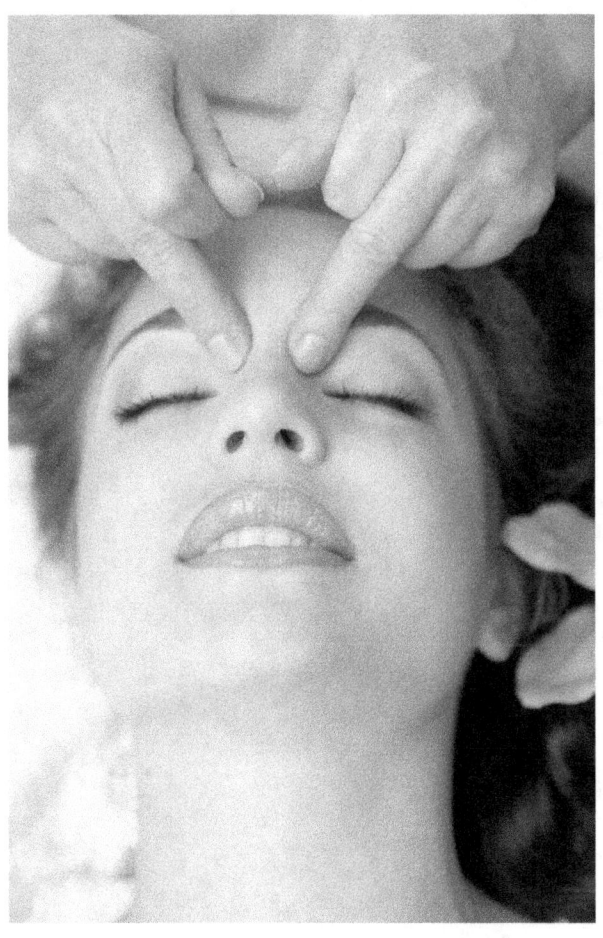

For Athletes

Blend:

- 2 tablespoons of coconut oil or other natural oil of your choice
- 2 drops of clove EO
- 2 drops of basil EO+
- 2 drops of rosemary EO

Add to your Epsom salt bath or use for self-massage. (focus on sore areas)

Easy Relax Sweet Mix

Blend:

- 2 tablespoons of coconut oil or other oil of your choice
- 2 drops of mandarin EO+
- 2 drop of mint EO+
- 2 drops of juniper EO+

Add to your Epsom salt bath or use for self-massage.

AROMATHERAPY PRECAUTIONS
Aromatherapy General Precautions

Aromatherapy is a very safe and easy therapy to use, but keep in mind that there are certain precautions:

- Remember to wash your hands after applying aromatherapy massage;

- Do not apply the essential oils in their pure form as they may cause an allergic reaction. Instead, use blends that contain 2-5% essential oils diluted in good-quality cold-pressed oil;

-After using citrus oils, like for example lemon, verbena, bergamot, orange etc. avoid direct sun exposure, even up to 8 hours after the treatment

- Do not apply oils after surgery (unless you have consulted with a doctor) or on open wounds or rashes of unknown origin;

- Do not use the oils after chemotherapy (unless suggested by a doctor);

- Keep the oils away from the eyes and mucus membranes;

- Use the oils only topically, do not ingest them (unless you are working with a certified scientific aromatherapist)

- Avoid rosemary, thyme, Spanish and common sage, fennel and hyssop if you suffer from high blood pressure;

- Do not apply the treatments described in this book on babies or infants. It doesn't mean that aromatherapy can never be used on babies and infants, but extremely low concentrations should be used. Always consult with a medical or naturopathy doctor first;

- After an aromatherapy massage always remember to wash your hands;

- Make sure that you research the brand, read safety instructions for each individual oil you buy/use and check the expiration date;

- Store your blends in dark glass bottles, preferably in a cool, dry and dark place and remember to use within a maximum of one month after mixing.

BONUS CHAPTER 2

How to Combine Epsom Salt with Mindfulness Meditation

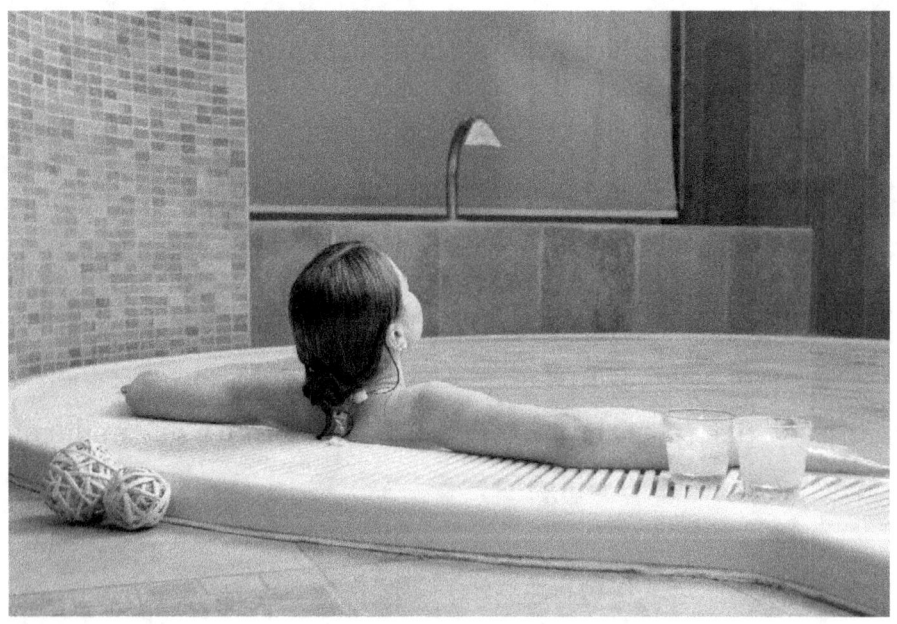

Here is something to think about and practice while enjoying your Epsom salt bath...Meditation is not only about spending hours on meditation cushions, you can practice it wherever you want, and it's always better if you feel relaxed (Epsom salt bath with essential oils is great for that).

Recent decades have seen a groundswell of research into the benefits of mindfulness meditation. Mindfulness's many benefits are now a part of general public knowledge and accepted scientific fact. Among these benefits are:

- deeper concentration and less tendency to distraction
- the ability to focus on the present moment
- an increase in nonjudgmental awareness
- the ability to see your emotions objectively
- letting go of outdated identities
- a general increase in positive emotions

How to practice mindfulness meditation

Practicing mindfulness meditation is quite simple and does not require a lot of preparation or training. Anyone can get into it. All you have to do is make a little time. *Learning how to do the practice is the practice.*

To begin with, set aside five to ten minutes of your day, every day. Find a quiet place to sit- a nice warm bath is great for that. Whatever works for you.

Your eyes can be open or closed; it's up to you. You may find that closing your eyes helps keep you from distraction, at least in the beginning.

The basic practice of sitting meditation is just to place your mind on the breath. *Mindfulness* in this context means being mindful of the breath, just following it as it moves in and out. When thoughts and sensations arise, you notice them and simply return your attention to the breath. It does not really matter what kind of thoughts or feelings come up. They could be boring thoughts about what you need to get from the store, or they could be mean, angry, happy, funny, creative, passionate—whatever.

Whatever comes up, just mentally label it *thinking* and return your attention to the breath. That's the nonjudgmental awareness we talked about earlier—whatever comes up, don't try to decide whether it's good or bad, don't accept or reject it. Just gently say to yourself, *Thinking*, and gently redirect your attention to the breath.

As you follow the breath in and out, you want to pay attention to the sensation of the breath—the feeling of the cool in-breath on your nostrils, and the warmth of the out-breath, the rise and fall of your lungs as you breathe in and out, whether the breath is long or short, shallow or deep, hard or gentle, and so on. In general, when meditating on the breath, you don't try to change the quality of the breath, but just let your lungs breathe however is most natural at any given time, and watch that.

Breathing is an effortless, autonomic function of the body, so we normally don't pay any attention to it. It just goes on in the background, all the time. In the practice of mindfulness, however, we don't take the breath for granted. Instead, we learn to appreciate the breath in its simplicity and variation. We develop a sense of wonder at something so simple and so necessary—taking in lungfuls of healthful, life-giving oxygen, which are delivered to the different organs of our body by the circulation of our blood. If we can learn to love and appreciate the simple fact of being alive, we can love ourselves.

When you begin meditating, it may seem that your discursive thoughts, the so-called "monkey mind," have only increased. Actually, nothing has increased; you just never noticed how active your mind is. Just stick with the practice of remaining mindful of the breath. Slowly, the speed of your thoughts will decrease. You will begin to notice and enjoy the vivid richness of the direct, sensory quality of your experience. This is the beginning of coming in touch with a quality of yourself that is fundamentally awake. It is the discovery of an innate source of goodness deep within your being.

Making friends with yourself

By breathing your awareness to the breath and learning to appreciate the simplicity of the present moment, you develop a sense of love for yourself that is not based on stories that you tell yourself, your wishes, likes and dislikes, who you tell yourself you want to be, negative thoughts, and so on. Instead, this newfound self-love is based on a direct, honest relationship to your own mind. This relationship is what has been called *making friends with yourself.*

The very act of meditation is an act of kindness to yourself. By setting aside time to rest and watch the breath, you are demonstrating a willingness and a commitment to sit with yourself quietly and gently. That is an act of compassion, a declaration of unconditional friendship to yourself and a willingness to get to know your own mind and heart more deeply.

It may sound strange to hear, but most of us do not really know ourselves that well. That's because we never take the time to get to know ourselves. So it's important to take that time, to slow down and rest. In this state of rest, we become more familiar with our own thoughts and feelings. Through the process of making friends with ourselves in meditation, we equip ourselves with self-love and self-compassion. Thus we can forgive ourselves when we make mistakes, or offer ourselves gentle encouragement and advice when we feel overwhelmed or anxious. This becomes a safeguard against the pessimism that attacks our motivation.

Deeper Concentration

It's easy to see how improving your concentration can increase your motivation to achieve your goals. In our daily lives, we're assailed from all sides by distractions and events vying for our attention. Meditation helps keep us on track by reducing the noise inside our heads. With more mindfulness, we will feel empowered to work towards our goals without going off track.

By bringing us into the present moment, mindfulness meditation helps induce a creative state of awareness psychologists call *flow*. Flow is full absorption in an activity with energetic focus and enjoyment. Research shows that mindfulness increases flow, focus, sharp thinking, self-control, and even the ability to meet deadlines.

Focus on the present moment

It's often helpful to clarify what you want for the future. If you know your desired outcome, that positive vision of the future can give you the energy that spurs you along on your journey to health and wellness you deserve.

Stress

A big part of stress is a physiological response in the body that psychologists call "fight or flight" mode. Stress is basically a response to something that your body and brain experience as a threat. So your heart rate increases, your muscles tense up, your breathing accelerates, blood pressure goes up, your digestive system is inhibited.

None of this is a problem if you're staring down a predator in the jungle. In fact, it's a good thing, because it gets you ready to either fight for your life, or run away very fast. And, in the wilderness, you'll need to do one of those things if you hope to live.

But in our hectic modern lives, it's often the case that what our brain experiences as a threat does not go away. So we stay in fight-or-flight for days, months, years. We can't sleep properly, often we don't feel like eating, and we're generally just miserable. Eventually it takes a big toll on our health and can lead to a number of diseases.

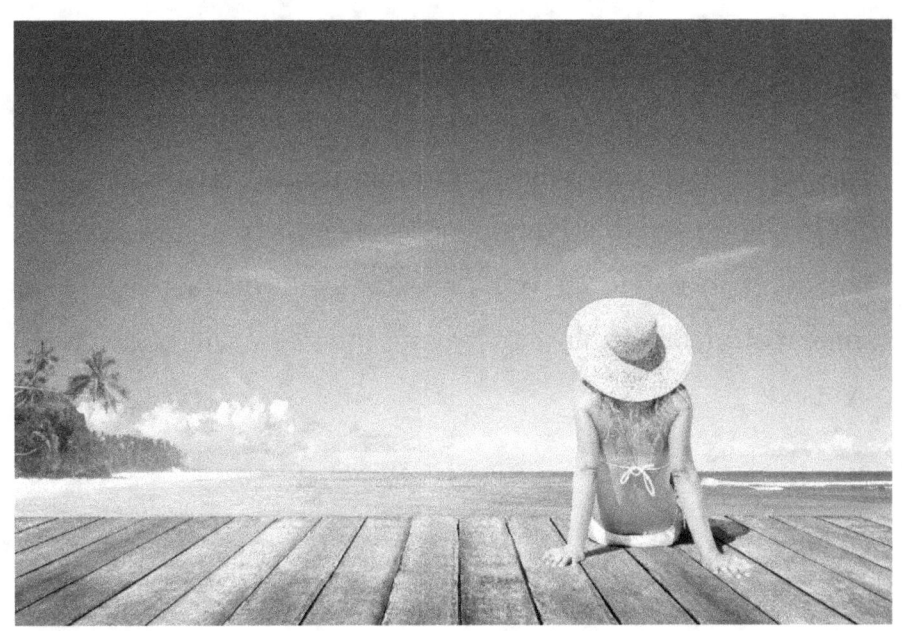

The good news is that meditation just by itself is shown to reduce stress very effectively. In addition to that, however, there are a few things you can do to bring your stress levels down. The most important thing to do is find ways to rest. Even if you are very busy, take some *me* time to just relax.

By "resting" I don't just mean sleeping, although that's important, too. I mean doing things that you find intrinsically enjoyable—that you don't have to force yourself to do, because you *want* to do them. That can be enjoying a tasty meal, talking a long walk in the afternoon, going for a swim, spending time with loved ones. Exercise is an excellent method for lowering stress, as is relaxing with friends and family.

The basic idea is that, since your brain thinks you are in danger, you need to do things that make the brain feel safe. You don't have to force your stress levels down. Just engage in some restful, enjoyable activity, and the stress will go down all by itself.

Healing from the inside out!

****

So....now you have reached the end of the fascinating journey into the world of Epsom Salt. Can you believe just how many uses it has? I hope by now you have been persuaded to add Epsom Salt to your shopping list and that you have already had your first Salt Spa in your very own bathroom. Whatever use you decide to put Epsom Salt to I hope you enjoy the experience and jeep this book to hand to check on quantities to use or to check for ideas.

Wishing you good health and a happy home!

Let's connect:

www.YourWellnessBooks.com

Free Complimentary eBook from Elena

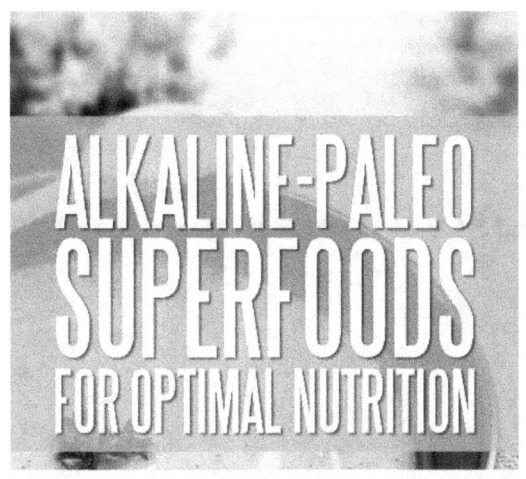

Free Sign Up Link:

www.YourWellnessBooks.com/newsletter

Problems with your download?

Contact us: elenajamesbooks@gmail.com

More Books by Elena Garcia

Available at:

www.YourWellnessBooks.com

www.ingramcontent.com/pod-product-compliance
Lightning Source LLC
Chambersburg PA
CBHW071749080526
44588CB00013B/2197